LOW-POTASSIUM RENAL DIET

COOKBOOK

Delicious and Nutritious Recipes for Kidney Health

Dr Lily Morgan

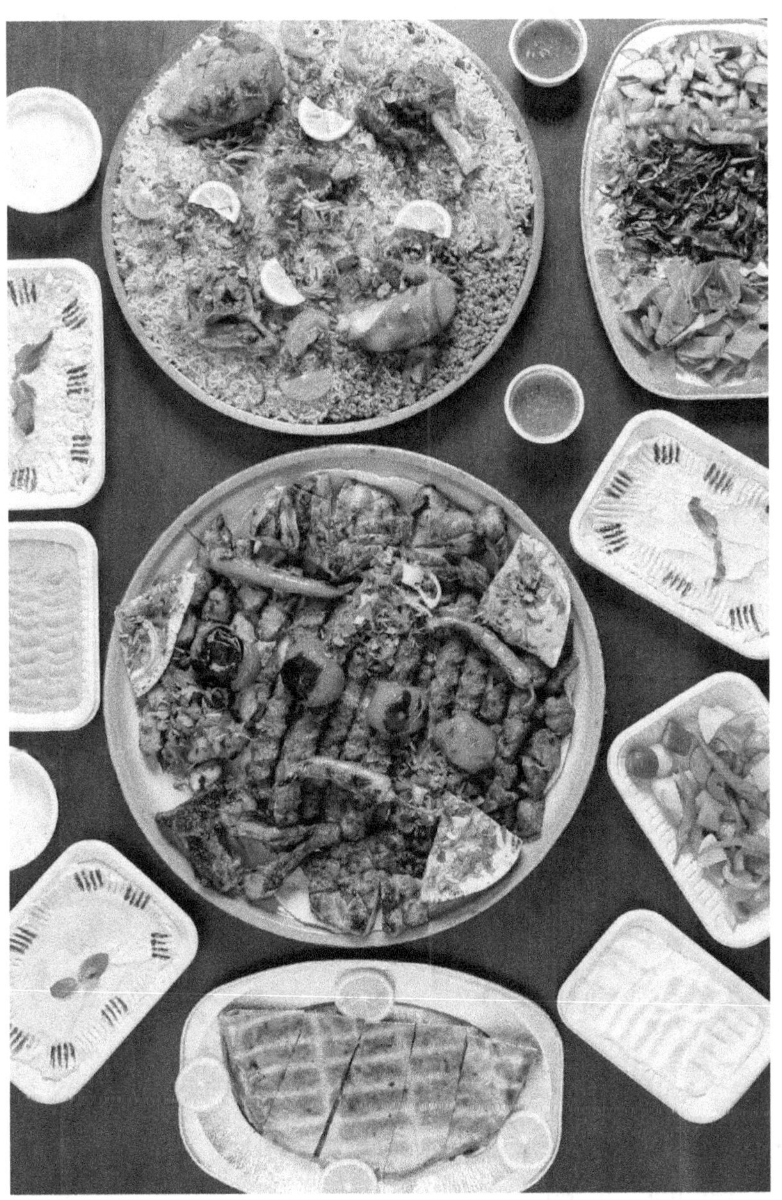

TABLE OF CONTENTS

Chapter 3: Lunch Recipes 38

Chapter 4: Dinner Recipes 54

Chapter 5: Snacks and Appetizers 74

Chapter 6: Desserts 88

INTRODUCTION

When it comes to embracing the Low-Potassium Renal Diet, knowledge is the first step towards success. This dietary approach is tailored to support individuals with kidney issues, specifically those who need to manage their potassium intake. Let's delve into the intricacies of understanding this diet, the profound benefits it offers, and some invaluable tips to thrive while adhering to it.

Understanding the Low-Potassium Renal Diet

At its core, the Low-Potassium Renal Diet is a specialized nutritional plan meticulously designed to safeguard the well-being of individuals with compromised kidney function. The kidneys, marvelous organs responsible for filtering out waste and excess nutrients, often face challenges when their function is impaired. In such cases, managing potassium intake becomes pivotal.

Potassium is a mineral found in many foods we consume daily. While it's essential for maintaining proper muscle and nerve function, excessive potassium can burden weakened kidneys. This diet, therefore, focuses on moderating potassium intake to alleviate stress on the kidneys and prevent potential complications.

Benefits of Following a Renal Diet

The benefits of embracing a Renal Diet extend far beyond the mere restriction of potassium. By adhering to this specialized dietary plan, individuals can experience a myriad of positive outcomes. Among these benefits are:

1. **Kidney Function Preservation:** A Renal Diet empowers individuals to safeguard and potentially improve their kidney function over time, providing a lifeline for those grappling with kidney-related issues.

2. **Blood Pressure Regulation**: This diet is inherently heart-friendly, helping to control blood pressure levels, a critical aspect of kidney health.

3. **Nutrient Optimization**: Renal Diet plans are crafted to ensure that essential nutrients are maintained at optimal levels, fostering overall well-being.

4. **Symptom Management:** It can alleviate symptoms associated with kidney disease, such as fluid retention and electrolyte imbalances, enhancing the quality of life.

Tips for Success on the Renal Diet

Embarking on the Renal Diet journey can initially appear challenging, but with the right guidance and mindset, success is within reach. Here are some practical tips to help you thrive on this dietary path:

1. **Portion Control:** Pay attention to portion sizes, as even low-potassium foods can pose challenges if consumed excessively.
2. **Diverse Choices:** Embrace variety in your diet. Explore different low-potassium foods to keep your meals interesting and nutritionally balanced.
3. **Read Labels:** Scrutinize food labels for potassium content, and opt for products with lower potassium levels.

4. **Fluid Management**: Monitor your fluid intake, as excessive fluids can strain the kidneys. Your dietitian can help you establish a suitable fluid intake limit.

5. **Medication Adherence**: If prescribed medications, take them as directed by your healthcare provider to support kidney function.

6. **Regular Monitoring**: Regularly monitor your kidney function with your healthcare team. This allows for timely adjustments to your dietary plan.

In summary, the Low-Potassium Renal Diet is not just a dietary regimen but a vital tool for managing kidney health. By understanding its principles, embracing its benefits, and following these success-oriented tips, individuals can take charge of their well-being, foster kidney health, and embark on a journey towards a healthier life.

Chapter 1: 30-Day Meal Plan

Week 1

Day 1:

- Breakfast: Low-Potassium Oatmeal
- Lunch: Chicken and Vegetable Stir-Fry
- Dinner: Baked Lemon Herb Chicken
- Snacks: Cucumber Slices with Hummus
- Dessert: Banana Ice Cream

Day 2:

- Breakfast: Spinach and Mushroom Scramble
- Lunch: Turkey and Avocado Wrap
- Dinner: Beef and Vegetable Stir-Fry
- Snacks: Guacamole and Salsa
- Dessert: Baked Apples

Day 3:

- Breakfast: Blueberry Pancakes
- Lunch: Quinoa Salad with Roasted Vegetables
- Dinner: Grilled Portobello Mushrooms

- Snacks: Baked Sweet Potato Fries
- Dessert: Chocolate Avocado Mousse

Day 4:

- Breakfast: Breakfast Burrito
- Lunch: Lentil Soup
- Dinner: Teriyaki Salmon
- Snacks: Popcorn with Herbs
- Dessert: Rice Pudding with Cinnamon

Day 5:

- Breakfast: Greek Yogurt Parfait
- Lunch: Tuna Salad Lettuce Wraps
- Dinner: Roasted Garlic and Herb Potatoes
- Snacks: Greek Yogurt Dip with Veggies
- Dessert: Berry Parfait

Day 6:

- Breakfast: Apple Cinnamon Muffins
- Lunch: Caprese Salad
- Dinner: Lemon Dill Tilapia
- Snacks: Rice Cakes with Almond Butter

- Dessert: Poached Pears

Day 7:

- Breakfast: Breakfast Quinoa Bowl
- Lunch: Vegetable and Rice Bowl
- Dinner: Ratatouille
- Snacks: Veggie Spring Rolls
- Dessert: Chia Seed Pudding

Week 2

Day 8:

- Breakfast: Avocado Toast
- Lunch: Egg Salad Sandwich
- Dinner: Pork Tenderloin with Apple Compote
- Snacks: Stuffed Mushrooms
- Dessert: Sorbet Trio

Day 9:

- Breakfast: Rice Pudding
- Lunch: Broccoli and Cheese Soup
- Dinner: Baked Cod with Herbed Quinoa
- Snacks: Cottage Cheese with Berries

- Dessert: Lemon Bars

Day 10:

- Breakfast: Veggie Omelette
- Lunch: Greek Salad with Grilled Chicken
- Dinner: Butternut Squash Risotto
- Snacks: Baked Parmesan Zucchini Chips
- Dessert: Pumpkin Pie Smoothie

Day 11:

- Breakfast: Banana Nut Smoothie
- Lunch: Chickpea and Spinach Salad
- Dinner: Lemon Rosemary Roasted Chicken
- Snacks: Fruit Kabobs
- Dessert: Strawberry Shortcake

Day 12:

- Breakfast: Creamy Polenta
- Lunch: Salmon and Asparagus
- Dinner: Sweet and Sour Tofu
- Snacks: Spinach Artichoke Dip
- Dessert: Oatmeal Raisin Cookies

Day 13:

- Breakfast: Sweet Potato Hash
- Lunch: Veggie Quesadilla
- Dinner: Zucchini Noodles with Pesto
- Snacks: Roasted Red Pepper and Walnut Dip
- Dessert: Mixed Berry Crisp

Day 14:

- Breakfast: Cottage Cheese Pancakes
- Lunch: Black Bean Soup
- Dinner: BBQ Pulled Chicken
- Snacks: Celery and Peanut Butter
- Dessert: Angel Food Cake with Berries

Week 3

Day 15:

- Breakfast: Spinach and Feta Frittata
- Lunch: Shrimp and Avocado Salad
- Dinner: Roasted Vegetable Lasagna
- Snacks: Edamame
- Dessert: Coconut Macaroons

Day 16:

- Breakfast: Cranberry Almond Oat Bars
- Lunch: Minestrone Soup
- Dinner: Spinach Stuffed Chicken
- Snacks: Caprese Skewers
- Dessert: Chocolate Covered Strawberries

Day 17:

- Breakfast: Peanut Butter Banana Toast
- Lunch: Roasted Red Pepper Hummus Wrap
- Dinner: Vegetable Curry with Brown Rice
- Snacks: Apple Slices with Cinnamon
- Dessert: Peach Cobbler

Day 18:

- Breakfast: Tomato Basil Bruschetta
- Lunch: Veggie and Brown Rice Stir-Fry
- Dinner: Baked Lemon Herb Chicken
- Snacks: Cucumber Slices with Hummus
- Dessert: Almond Joy Bites

Day 19:

- Breakfast: Greek Yogurt Parfait
- Lunch: Turkey and Avocado Wrap
- Dinner: Beef and Vegetable Stir-Fry
- Snacks: Guacamole and Salsa
- Dessert: Baked Apples

Day 20:

- Breakfast: Apple Cinnamon Muffins
- Lunch: Quinoa Salad with Roasted Vegetables
- Dinner: Grilled Portobello Mushrooms
- Snacks: Baked Sweet Potato Fries
- Dessert: Chocolate Avocado Mousse

Day 21:

- Breakfast: Breakfast Quinoa Bowl
- Lunch: Lentil Soup
- Dinner: Teriyaki Salmon
- Snacks: Popcorn with Herbs
- Dessert: Rice Pudding with Cinnamon

Week 4

Day 22:

- Breakfast: Avocado Toast
- Lunch: Egg Salad Sandwich
- Dinner: Pork Tenderloin with Apple Compote
- Snacks: Stuffed Mushrooms
- Dessert: Sorbet Trio

Day 23:

- Breakfast: Rice Pudding
- Lunch: Broccoli and Cheese Soup
- Dinner: Baked Cod with Herbed Quinoa
- Snacks: Cottage Cheese with Berries
- Dessert: Lemon Bars

Day 24:

- Breakfast: Veggie Omelette
- Lunch: Greek Salad with Grilled Chicken
- Dinner: Butternut Squash Risotto
- Snacks: Baked Parmesan Zucchini Chips
- Dessert: Pumpkin Pie Smoothie

Day 25:

- Breakfast: Banana Nut Smoothie
- Lunch: Chickpea and Spinach Salad
- Dinner: Lemon Rosemary Roasted Chicken
- Snacks: Fruit Kabobs
- Dessert: Strawberry Shortcake

Day 26:

- Breakfast: Creamy Polenta
- Lunch: Salmon and Asparagus
- Dinner: Sweet and Sour Tofu
- Snacks: Spinach Artichoke Dip
- Dessert: Oatmeal Raisin Cookies

Day 27:

- Breakfast: Sweet Potato Hash
- Lunch: Veggie Quesadilla
- Dinner: Zucchini Noodles with Pesto
- Snacks: Roasted Red Pepper and Walnut Dip
- Dessert: Mixed Berry Crisp

Day 28:

- Breakfast: Cottage Cheese Pancakes
- Lunch: Black Bean Soup
- Dinner: BBQ Pulled Chicken
- Snacks: Celery and Peanut Butter
- Dessert: Angel Food Cake with Berries

Day 29:

- Breakfast: Spinach and Feta Frittata
- Lunch: Shrimp and Avocado Salad
- Dinner: Roasted Vegetable Lasagna
- Snacks: Edamame
- Dessert: Coconut Macaroons

Day 30:

- Breakfast: Cranberry Almond Oat Bars
- Lunch: Minestrone Soup
- Dinner: Spinach Stuffed Chicken
- Snacks: Caprese Skewers
- Dessert: Chocolate Covered Strawberries

Congratulations on completing your 30-day meal plan! Continue to adapt and enjoy these delicious low-potassium renal diet recipes while keeping in mind your dietary requirements and preferences.

Chapter 2: Breakfast Recipes

In the realm of Chapter 2, the dawn brings a splendid array of Breakfast Recipes that will ignite your taste buds and nourish your body. From the comforting warmth of Low-Potassium Oatmeal to the zest of Tomato Basil Bruschetta, this chapter promises a flavorful journey through the most important meal of the day.

Low-Potassium Oatmeal

Ingredients:

- 1/2 cup rolled oats
- 1 cup unsweetened almond milk
- 1 small banana, sliced
- 1 tablespoon honey
- 1/4 teaspoon cinnamon
- Chopped almonds (optional)

Instructions:

1. Combine oats and almond milk in a saucepan.

2. Heat over medium heat, stirring occasionally, until oats are cooked and mixture thickens.

3. Top with banana slices, drizzle with honey, sprinkle cinnamon, and add chopped almonds if desired.

Spinach and Mushroom Scramble

Ingredients:

- 2 eggs
- 1/4 cup spinach, chopped
- 1/4 cup mushrooms, sliced
- Salt and pepper to taste
- Cooking spray

Instructions:

1. In a bowl, beat eggs and season with salt and pepper.
2. Heat a non-stick skillet over medium heat, lightly coat with cooking spray.
3. Add mushrooms and spinach, sauté until tender.
4. Pour beaten eggs over the veggies, cook, and stir until scrambled.

Blueberry Pancakes

Ingredients:

- 1/2 cup whole wheat flour
- 1/2 teaspoon baking powder
- 1/2 cup blueberries
- 1/4 cup unsweetened almond milk
- 1 egg
- 1 tablespoon honey
- Cooking spray

Instructions:

1. In a bowl, combine flour and baking powder.
2. In another bowl, whisk together almond milk, egg, and honey.
3. Pour wet ingredients into dry, stir until just combined.
4. Fold in blueberries.
5. Heat a skillet, coat with cooking spray, and pour batter to make pancakes.

Breakfast Burrito

Ingredients:

- 2 eggs
- 2 small whole-wheat tortillas
- 1/4 cup black beans, drained and rinsed
- 1/4 cup salsa
- 1/4 cup avocado, diced
- Salt and pepper to taste

Instructions:

1. Scramble the eggs in a pan.
2. Warm tortillas in the microwave.
3. Assemble by placing eggs, black beans, salsa, and avocado on each tortilla.
4. Season with salt and pepper, then roll up into burritos.

Greek Yogurt Parfait

Ingredients:

- 1 cup Greek yogurt

- 1/2 cup mixed berries (strawberries, blueberries, raspberries)
- 2 tablespoons honey
- 1/4 cup granola

Instructions:

1. In a glass, layer Greek yogurt, mixed berries, and honey.
2. Top with granola for added crunch.

Apple Cinnamon Muffins

Ingredients:

- 1 cup oat flour
- 1 teaspoon baking powder
- 1/2 teaspoon cinnamon
- 1/4 cup unsweetened applesauce
- 1/4 cup almond milk
- 1 egg
- 1/4 cup diced apples

Instructions:

1. Preheat oven to 350°F (175°C) and line a muffin tin.

2. In a bowl, combine oat flour, baking powder, and cinnamon.

3. In another bowl, mix applesauce, almond milk, and egg.

4. Combine wet and dry ingredients, then fold in diced apples.

5. Pour batter into muffin cups and bake for 20-25 minutes.

Breakfast Quinoa Bowl

Ingredients:

- 1/2 cup cooked quinoa
- 1/4 cup sliced almonds
- 1/2 cup mixed berries
- 1 tablespoon honey
- 1/4 teaspoon vanilla extract

Instructions:

1. In a bowl, combine quinoa, sliced almonds, and mixed berries.

2. Drizzle with honey and vanilla extract.

Avocado Toast

Ingredients:

- 2 slices whole-grain bread
- 1 ripe avocado
- Salt and pepper to taste
- Red pepper flakes (optional)

Instructions:

1. Toast the bread.
2. Mash the ripe avocado and spread it onto the toasted bread.
3. Season with salt, pepper, and red pepper flakes if desired.

Rice Pudding

Ingredients:

- 1/2 cup cooked rice
- 1 cup unsweetened almond milk
- 1 tablespoon honey
- 1/4 teaspoon vanilla extract
- Ground cinnamon for garnish

Instructions:

1. In a saucepan, combine rice, almond milk, honey, and vanilla extract.
2. Heat over low heat, stirring until thickened.
3. Serve warm or chilled, sprinkled with ground cinnamon.

Veggie Omelette

Ingredients:

- 2 eggs
- 1/4 cup diced bell peppers (any color)
- 1/4 cup diced tomatoes
- 1/4 cup diced onions
- Salt and pepper to taste
- Cooking spray

Instructions:

1. In a bowl, whisk eggs and season with salt and pepper.
2. Heat a non-stick skillet over medium heat, coat with cooking spray.
3. Add diced vegetables and sauté until tender.

4. Pour beaten eggs over the veggies, cook until set, then fold in half.

Banana Nut Smoothie

Ingredients:

- 1 ripe banana
- 1/2 cup unsweetened almond milk
- 1 tablespoon almond butter
- 1/2 teaspoon cinnamon
- 1 tablespoon chopped nuts (e.g., almonds, walnuts)

Instructions:

1. In a blender, combine banana, almond milk, almond butter, and cinnamon.
2. Blend until smooth.
3. Top with chopped nuts for added crunch.

Creamy Polenta

Ingredients:

- 1/2 cup cornmeal
- 1 1/2 cups water

- 1/4 cup grated Parmesan cheese
- Salt and pepper to taste

Instructions:

1. In a saucepan, bring water to a boil.
2. Slowly whisk in cornmeal, stirring constantly.
3. Cook over low heat, stirring until thickened.
4. Remove from heat, stir in Parmesan cheese, salt, and pepper.

Sweet Potato Hash

Ingredients:

- 1 sweet potato, diced
- 1/4 cup diced onions
- 1/4 cup diced bell peppers (any color)
- 1/4 teaspoon paprika
- Salt and pepper to taste
- Cooking spray

Instructions:

1. Heat a skillet over medium heat, coat with cooking spray.

2. Add sweet potato, onions, and bell peppers.

3. Sprinkle with paprika, salt, and pepper.

4. Sauté until sweet potatoes are tender and lightly browned.

Cottage Cheese Pancakes

Ingredients:

- 1/2 cup cottage cheese
- 2 eggs
- 1/4 cup oat flour
- 1/2 teaspoon vanilla extract
- Cooking spray

Instructions:

1. In a blender, combine cottage cheese, eggs, oat flour, and vanilla extract.

2. Blend until smooth.

3. Heat a skillet over medium heat, coat with cooking spray.

4. Pour batter to make pancakes.

Spinach and Feta Frittata

Ingredients:

- 2 eggs
- 1/4 cup chopped spinach
- 2 tablespoons crumbled feta cheese
- Salt and pepper to taste
- Cooking spray

Instructions:

1. In a bowl, beat eggs and season with salt and pepper.
2. Heat a non-stick skillet over medium heat, coat with cooking spray.
3. Add chopped spinach and feta cheese.
4. Pour beaten eggs over the mixture, cook until set.

Cranberry Almond Oat Bars

Ingredients:

- 1 cup rolled oats
- 1/4 cup dried cranberries
- 1/4 cup chopped almonds
- 2 tablespoons honey

- 1/4 cup unsweetened applesauce

Instructions:

1. Preheat oven to 350°F (175°C) and grease a baking dish.
2. In a bowl, mix oats, cranberries, and almonds.
3. In another bowl, combine honey and applesauce.
4. Combine wet and dry ingredients, then press into the baking dish.
5. Bake for 20-25 minutes until golden.

Peanut Butter Banana Toast

Ingredients:

- 2 slices whole-grain bread
- 2 tablespoons peanut butter
- 1 banana, sliced
- Honey for drizzling

Instructions:

1. Toast the bread.
2. Spread peanut butter on the toasted bread.
3. Top with banana slices and drizzle with honey.

Tomato Basil Bruschetta

Ingredients:

- 2 slices whole-grain bread
- 2 ripe tomatoes, diced
- 1/4 cup fresh basil leaves, chopped
- 1 clove garlic, minced
- 1 tablespoon olive oil
- Balsamic glaze (optional)

Instructions:

1. Toast the bread.
2. In a bowl, combine diced tomatoes, chopped basil, minced garlic, and olive oil.
3. Spoon the tomato mixture onto the toasted bread.
4. Optionally, drizzle with balsamic glaze for extra flavor.

Chapter 3: Lunch Recipes

In this chapter, you'll discover a delightful array of lunch recipes that are both satisfying and nutritionally balanced. These dishes are carefully crafted to fit within the guidelines of a low-potassium renal diet, ensuring you enjoy your midday meals while prioritizing your kidney health.

Chicken and Vegetable Stir-Fry

Ingredients:

- 1 boneless, skinless chicken breast, sliced
- 1 cup broccoli florets
- 1 red bell pepper, sliced
- 1 cup snap peas
- 2 tablespoons low-sodium soy sauce
- 1 teaspoon sesame oil
- 1 teaspoon minced garlic
- 1 teaspoon minced ginger
- 1 tablespoon olive oil

Instructions:

1. Heat olive oil in a skillet over medium-high heat.

2. Add chicken and stir-fry until cooked through.

3. Remove chicken from the skillet.

4. In the same skillet, add garlic, ginger, and vegetables. Stir-fry for a few minutes.

5. Return the cooked chicken to the skillet, add soy sauce and sesame oil. Cook until heated through.

Turkey and Avocado Wrap

Ingredients:

- 4 large lettuce leaves
- 8 oz lean turkey slices
- 1 ripe avocado, sliced
- 1/2 cup diced tomatoes
- 1/4 cup sliced red onion
- 2 tablespoons Greek yogurt
- 1 tablespoon lemon juice
- Salt and pepper to taste

Instructions:

1. Lay out lettuce leaves.

2. Divide turkey, avocado, tomatoes, and red onion evenly among the leaves.

3. In a small bowl, mix Greek yogurt, lemon juice, salt, and pepper.

4. Drizzle the yogurt dressing over each wrap, then roll them up.

Quinoa Salad with Roasted Vegetables

Ingredients:

- 1 cup quinoa, cooked and cooled
- 1 cup roasted vegetables (e.g., bell peppers, zucchini, and eggplant)
- 1/4 cup chopped fresh parsley
- 2 tablespoons olive oil
- 2 tablespoons balsamic vinegar
- Salt and pepper to taste

Instructions:

1. In a large bowl, combine quinoa, roasted vegetables, and chopped parsley.

2. In a separate bowl, whisk together olive oil and balsamic vinegar.

3. Pour the dressing over the salad and toss to coat.

4. Season with salt and pepper.

Lentil Soup

Ingredients:

- 1 cup green or brown lentils, rinsed
- 1 onion, chopped
- 2 carrots, diced
- 2 celery stalks, diced
- 4 cups low-sodium vegetable broth
- 1 teaspoon dried thyme
- 1 bay leaf
- Salt and pepper to taste

Instructions:

1. In a large pot, sauté onions, carrots, and celery until they start to soften.

2. Add lentils, vegetable broth, thyme, and bay leaf.

3. Bring to a boil, then reduce heat and simmer for 30-40 minutes until lentils are tender.

4. Season with salt and pepper.

Tuna Salad Lettuce Wraps

Ingredients:

- 1 can (5 oz) low-sodium tuna, drained
- 2 tablespoons Greek yogurt
- 1 tablespoon lemon juice
- 1/4 cup diced celery
- 1/4 cup diced red onion
- 1/4 cup chopped fresh parsley
- Lettuce leaves for wrapping

Instructions:

1. In a bowl, combine tuna, Greek yogurt, lemon juice, celery, red onion, and parsley.
2. Mix until well combined.
3. Spoon the tuna salad into lettuce leaves and wrap them up.

Caprese Salad

Ingredients:

- 2 ripe tomatoes, sliced
- 4 oz fresh mozzarella cheese, sliced
- Fresh basil leaves
- 2 tablespoons balsamic vinegar
- 2 tablespoons olive oil
- Salt and pepper to taste

Instructions:

1. Arrange tomato and mozzarella slices on a plate, alternating them.
2. Tuck fresh basil leaves between the slices.
3. Drizzle with balsamic vinegar and olive oil.
4. Season with salt and pepper.

Vegetable and Rice Bowl

Ingredients:

- 1 cup cooked brown rice
- 1 cup mixed steamed vegetables (e.g., broccoli, carrots, and snap peas)

- 1/4 cup sliced almonds

- 2 tablespoons low-sodium soy sauce

- 1 teaspoon sesame seeds

Instructions:

1. Place cooked rice in a bowl.

2. Top with steamed vegetables and sliced almonds.

3. Drizzle with soy sauce and sprinkle sesame seeds.

Egg Salad Sandwich

Ingredients:

- 4 hard-boiled eggs, chopped

- 1/4 cup Greek yogurt

- 1 tablespoon Dijon mustard

- 2 tablespoons chopped fresh chives

- Salt and pepper to taste

- Whole-grain bread or lettuce leaves for serving

Instructions:

1. In a bowl, combine chopped hard-boiled eggs, Greek yogurt, Dijon mustard, and chives.

2. Mix until well combined.

3. Season with salt and pepper.

4. Serve as a sandwich with whole-grain bread or as lettuce wraps.

Broccoli and Cheese Soup

Ingredients:

- 2 cups steamed broccoli florets
- 2 cups low-sodium vegetable broth
- 1 cup shredded low-sodium cheddar cheese
- 1/2 cup diced onion
- 2 cloves garlic, minced
- 1/2 cup Greek yogurt
- Salt and pepper to taste

Instructions:

1. In a pot, sauté onions and garlic until softened.

2. Add steamed broccoli and vegetable broth. Simmer for 10-15 minutes.

3. Use an immersion blender to puree the soup.

4. Return to low heat and stir in cheddar cheese until melted.

5. Mix in Greek yogurt and season with salt and pepper.

Greek Salad with Grilled Chicken

Ingredients:

- 2 boneless, skinless chicken breasts
- 1 cucumber, sliced
- 1 cup cherry tomatoes, halved
- 1/2 red onion, thinly sliced
- 1/2 cup Kalamata olives
- 4 oz feta cheese, crumbled
- Greek dressing (olive oil, lemon juice, oregano, salt, and pepper)

Instructions:

1. Grill chicken breasts until cooked through, then slice.
2. In a large bowl, combine cucumber, cherry tomatoes, red onion, Kalamata olives, and feta cheese.
3. Drizzle with Greek dressing.
4. Top with grilled chicken slices.

Chickpea and Spinach Salad

Ingredients:

- 1 can (15 oz) chickpeas, drained and rinsed

- 2 cups fresh spinach leaves
- 1/4 cup diced red bell pepper
- 1/4 cup diced cucumber
- 2 tablespoons olive oil
- 1 tablespoon lemon juice
- 1 teaspoon minced garlic
- Salt and pepper to taste

Instructions:

1. In a large bowl, combine chickpeas, spinach, red bell pepper, and cucumber.
2. In a separate bowl, whisk together olive oil, lemon juice, minced garlic, salt, and pepper.
3. Drizzle the dressing over the salad and toss to coat.

Salmon and Asparagus

Ingredients:

- 2 salmon fillets
- 1 bunch of asparagus
- 2 tablespoons olive oil
- Lemon zest and juice
- Fresh dill (optional)

- Salt and pepper to taste

Instructions:

1. Preheat your oven to 400°F (200°C).
2. Place salmon fillets on a baking sheet and arrange asparagus around them.
3. Drizzle olive oil over both salmon and asparagus.
4. Sprinkle with lemon zest, lemon juice, fresh dill (if desired), salt, and pepper.
5. Bake for 15-20 minutes or until salmon flakes easily with a fork.

Veggie Quesadilla

Ingredients:

- Whole-wheat tortillas
- 1 cup diced bell peppers (various colors)
- 1/2 cup diced red onion
- 1/2 cup black beans, drained and rinsed
- 1/2 cup shredded low-sodium cheese
- 1 teaspoon olive oil
- Salsa (optional)

Instructions:

1. In a pan, heat olive oil over medium heat.

2. Add bell peppers and red onion, sauté until softened.

3. Place a tortilla in the pan, sprinkle with cheese, add sautéed veggies and black beans, then top with another tortilla.

4. Cook until the cheese is melted and the tortilla is crispy.

5. Cut into wedges and serve with salsa if desired.

Black Bean Soup

Ingredients:

- 2 cans (15 oz each) low-sodium black beans, drained and rinsed
- 1 onion, chopped
- 2 cloves garlic, minced
- 1 teaspoon cumin
- 1 teaspoon chili powder
- 4 cups low-sodium vegetable broth
- Salt and pepper to taste

Instructions:

1. In a pot, sauté onions and garlic until fragrant.
2. Add black beans, cumin, chili powder, and vegetable broth.
3. Bring to a boil, then reduce heat and simmer for 20-30 minutes.
4. Use an immersion blender to puree the soup.
5. Season with salt and pepper.

Shrimp and Avocado Salad

Ingredients:

- 8 oz cooked shrimp, peeled and deveined
- 1 ripe avocado, diced
- 1/2 cup cherry tomatoes, halved
- 1/4 cup diced red onion
- Fresh cilantro leaves
- Lime juice
- Salt and pepper to taste

Instructions:

1. In a bowl, combine cooked shrimp, diced avocado, cherry tomatoes, and red onion.

2. Drizzle with lime juice.

3. Garnish with fresh cilantro leaves.

4. Season with salt and pepper.

Minestrone Soup

Ingredients:

- 1 cup low-sodium vegetable broth
- 1 can (15 oz) low-sodium diced tomatoes
- 1/2 cup cooked kidney beans
- 1/2 cup diced zucchini
- 1/2 cup diced carrots
- 1/2 cup cooked whole wheat pasta
- 1 teaspoon dried basil
- 1 teaspoon dried oregano
- Salt and pepper to taste

Instructions:

1. In a pot, combine vegetable broth, diced tomatoes, kidney beans, zucchini, carrots, and cooked pasta.

2. Add dried basil and oregano.

3. Bring to a simmer and cook for 15-20 minutes.

4. Season with salt and pepper.

Roasted Red Pepper Hummus Wrap

Ingredients:

- Whole-grain tortilla
- 1/4 cup roasted red pepper hummus
- 1/2 cup mixed greens
- 1/4 cup sliced cucumber
- 1/4 cup sliced red bell pepper
- 1/4 cup sliced black olives
- Feta cheese crumbles (optional)

Instructions:

1. Spread hummus evenly on a whole-grain tortilla.
2. Layer with mixed greens, sliced cucumber, red bell pepper, and black olives.
3. Add feta cheese crumbles if desired.
4. Roll up the tortilla and cut in half.

Veggie and Brown Rice Stir-Fry

Ingredients:

- 1 cup cooked brown rice

- 1 cup mixed stir-fry vegetables (e.g., broccoli, carrots, and bell peppers)
- 2 tablespoons low-sodium soy sauce
- 1 teaspoon sesame oil
- 1/2 teaspoon minced garlic
- 1/2 teaspoon minced ginger
- 1 tablespoon olive oil

Instructions:

1. Heat olive oil in a pan over medium-high heat.
2. Add garlic and ginger, sauté for a minute.
3. Add stir-fry vegetables and cook until tender-crisp.
4. Stir in cooked brown rice, soy sauce, and sesame oil.
5. Cook until heated through.

Chapter 4: Dinner Recipes

In this chapter, we delve into a delightful array of dinner recipes that not only cater to your dietary needs but also burst with flavors that will leave your taste buds satisfied. From succulent meats to hearty vegetarian options, you'll find something to suit every palate.

Baked Lemon Herb Chicken

Ingredients:

- 4 boneless, skinless chicken breasts
- 2 tablespoons olive oil
- 1 lemon, juiced and zested
- 2 cloves garlic, minced
- 1 teaspoon dried rosemary
- Salt and pepper to taste

Instructions:

1. Preheat your oven to 375°F (190°C).
2. In a bowl, mix together olive oil, lemon juice, lemon zest, minced garlic, rosemary, salt, and pepper.

3. Place chicken breasts in a baking dish and pour the lemon herb mixture over them.

4. Bake for 25-30 minutes or until the chicken is cooked through and no longer pink in the center.

Beef and Vegetable Stir-Fry

Ingredients:

- 1 pound beef sirloin, thinly sliced
- 2 cups broccoli florets
- 1 red bell pepper, sliced
- 1 cup snap peas
- 3 cloves garlic, minced
- 2 tablespoons soy sauce
- 1 tablespoon vegetable oil
- 1 teaspoon sesame oil

Instructions:

1. Heat vegetable oil in a large skillet or wok over high heat.

2. Add beef slices and stir-fry until browned, then remove from the pan.

3. In the same pan, add garlic, broccoli, red bell pepper, and snap peas. Stir-fry for a few minutes until the vegetables are tender-crisp.

4. Return the beef to the pan, add soy sauce and sesame oil, and toss to combine. Cook for another minute.

5. Serve hot with steamed rice.

Grilled Portobello Mushrooms

Ingredients:

- 4 large Portobello mushrooms
- 2 tablespoons olive oil
- 2 cloves garlic, minced
- 1 teaspoon dried thyme
- Salt and pepper to taste

Instructions:

1. Preheat your grill to medium-high heat.

2. Clean the mushrooms and remove the stems.

3. In a small bowl, mix olive oil, minced garlic, dried thyme, salt, and pepper.

4. Brush the mushroom caps with the olive oil mixture.

5. Grill the mushrooms for 4-5 minutes on each side, or until they are tender.

Teriyaki Salmon

Ingredients:

- 4 salmon fillets
- 1/2 cup teriyaki sauce
- 2 tablespoons brown sugar
- 2 cloves garlic, minced
- 1 teaspoon grated ginger
- 1 tablespoon sesame seeds

Instructions:

1. In a small saucepan, combine teriyaki sauce, brown sugar, minced garlic, and grated ginger. Bring to a simmer and cook for 5 minutes until the sauce thickens.
2. Preheat your grill or broiler.
3. Brush the salmon fillets with the teriyaki sauce mixture and grill or broil for about 5-7 minutes on each side, or until the salmon flakes easily.
4. Sprinkle with sesame seeds before serving.

Roasted Garlic and Herb Potatoes

Ingredients:

- 4 cups baby potatoes, halved
- 2 tablespoons olive oil
- 4 cloves garlic, minced
- 1 teaspoon dried thyme
- Salt and pepper to taste

Instructions:

1. Preheat your oven to 400°F (200°C).
2. In a large bowl, toss the halved baby potatoes with olive oil, minced garlic, dried thyme, salt, and pepper.
3. Spread the potatoes in a single layer on a baking sheet.
4. Roast in the oven for about 30-35 minutes, or until the potatoes are golden brown and tender, stirring occasionally.

Lemon Dill Tilapia

Ingredients:

- 4 tilapia fillets
- 2 tablespoons olive oil
- 2 tablespoons fresh lemon juice
- 2 teaspoons dried dill
- Salt and pepper to taste
- Lemon wedges for garnish

Instructions:

1. Preheat your oven to 375°F (190°C).
2. In a small bowl, mix olive oil, lemon juice, dried dill, salt, and pepper.
3. Place tilapia fillets on a baking dish and drizzle with the lemon dill mixture.
4. Bake for 15-20 minutes, or until the tilapia is cooked through and flakes easily.
5. Serve with lemon wedges for added zest.

Ratatouille

Ingredients:

- 1 eggplant, diced
- 1 zucchini, sliced
- 1 yellow bell pepper, sliced
- 1 red onion, sliced
- 2 cloves garlic, minced
- 1 can (14 oz) diced tomatoes
- 2 tablespoons olive oil
- 1 teaspoon dried basil
- 1 teaspoon dried thyme
- Salt and pepper to taste

Instructions:

1. Heat olive oil in a large skillet over medium heat.
2. Add minced garlic, eggplant, zucchini, yellow bell pepper, and red onion. Sauté for about 5-7 minutes until the vegetables start to soften.
3. Stir in the diced tomatoes, dried basil, dried thyme, salt, and pepper.
4. Cover and simmer for 15-20 minutes until the vegetables are tender.

Pork Tenderloin with Apple Compote

Ingredients:

- 2 pork tenderloins
- 2 tablespoons olive oil
- 2 apples, peeled, cored, and sliced
- 1/4 cup brown sugar
- 1/2 teaspoon ground cinnamon
- Salt and pepper to taste

Instructions:

1. Preheat your oven to 375°F (190°C).
2. Season pork tenderloins with salt and pepper.
3. In a large ovenproof skillet, heat olive oil over medium-high heat. Add the pork tenderloins and sear until browned on all sides.
4. In a separate saucepan, combine sliced apples, brown sugar, and ground cinnamon. Cook over medium heat until apples are tender and the mixture thickens.
5. Spread the apple compote over the pork tenderloins in the skillet.

6. Transfer the skillet to the oven and roast for 20-25 minutes, or until the pork reaches an internal temperature of 145°F (63°C).

Baked Cod with Herbed Quinoa

Ingredients:

- 4 cod fillets
- 1 cup quinoa, rinsed and drained
- 2 cups chicken or vegetable broth
- 2 tablespoons fresh parsley, chopped
- 2 tablespoons fresh dill, chopped
- 1 lemon, sliced
- Salt and pepper to taste

Instructions:

1. Preheat your oven to 375°F (190°C).
2. In a saucepan, bring the chicken or vegetable broth to a boil. Add quinoa, reduce heat, cover, and simmer for 15-20 minutes, or until quinoa is tender.
3. Season cod fillets with salt and pepper and place them on a baking dish.

4. In a bowl, combine cooked quinoa, fresh parsley, and fresh dill. Spoon the quinoa mixture over the cod fillets.

5. Top each fillet with a lemon slice.

6. Bake for 20-25 minutes, or until the cod flakes easily with a fork.

Butternut Squash Risotto

Ingredients:

- 2 cups Arborio rice
- 4 cups low-sodium vegetable broth
- 2 cups diced butternut squash
- 1 small onion, finely chopped
- 2 cloves garlic, minced
- 1/2 cup grated Parmesan cheese
- 2 tablespoons olive oil
- Salt and pepper to taste

Instructions:

1. In a large skillet, heat olive oil over medium heat. Add chopped onion and garlic and sauté until translucent.

2. Add Arborio rice and cook, stirring constantly, for about 2 minutes until it's lightly toasted.

3. Gradually add vegetable broth, one ladle at a time, stirring until the liquid is absorbed before adding more.

4. Stir in diced butternut squash and continue to cook and stir until the rice is creamy and the squash is tender.

5. Remove from heat and stir in grated Parmesan cheese.

6. Season with salt and pepper to taste before serving.

Lemon Rosemary Roasted Chicken

Ingredients:

- 4 bone-in, skin-on chicken thighs
- 2 tablespoons olive oil
- 2 lemons, juiced and zested
- 2 cloves garlic, minced
- 2 teaspoons dried rosemary
- Salt and pepper to taste
- Fresh rosemary sprigs for garnish

Instructions:

1. Preheat your oven to 375°F (190°C).

2. In a bowl, combine olive oil, lemon juice, lemon zest, minced garlic, dried rosemary, salt, and pepper.

3. Place chicken thighs in a baking dish and pour the lemon rosemary mixture over them.

4. Roast in the oven for 35-40 minutes, or until the chicken is cooked through and the skin is golden and crispy.

5. Garnish with fresh rosemary sprigs before serving.

Sweet and Sour Tofu

Ingredients:

- 1 block of extra-firm tofu, cubed
- 1 bell pepper, sliced
- 1 onion, sliced
- 1/4 cup rice vinegar
- 2 tablespoons soy sauce
- 2 tablespoons brown sugar
- 1 tablespoon cornstarch
- 1/4 cup pineapple chunks
- 1 tablespoon vegetable oil

Instructions:

1. In a small bowl, whisk together rice vinegar, soy sauce, brown sugar, and cornstarch to make the sweet and sour sauce.

2. Heat vegetable oil in a large skillet over medium-high heat. Add tofu cubes and cook until they are golden and crispy on all sides. Remove tofu from the skillet.

3. In the same skillet, add sliced bell pepper and onion and sauté until they start to soften.

4. Return tofu to the skillet and pour the sweet and sour sauce over it. Add pineapple chunks.

5. Cook for a few more minutes until the sauce thickens and coats the tofu and vegetables.

Zucchini Noodles with Pesto

Ingredients:

- 4 medium zucchinis, spiralized into noodles
- 1/2 cup basil pesto
- 1/4 cup grated Parmesan cheese
- Cherry tomatoes for garnish
- Salt and pepper to taste

Instructions:

1. Heat a large skillet over medium heat.
2. Add zucchini noodles and cook for about 2-3 minutes, or until they are tender but not mushy.
3. Toss the zucchini noodles with basil pesto and grated Parmesan cheese.
4. Season with salt and pepper to taste.
5. Garnish with halved cherry tomatoes before serving.

BBQ Pulled Chicken

Ingredients:

- 4 boneless, skinless chicken breasts
- 1 cup low-sodium barbecue sauce
- 1/2 cup chicken broth
- 1/4 cup brown sugar
- 1 teaspoon paprika
- 1/2 teaspoon garlic powder
- 1/2 teaspoon onion powder
- Salt and pepper to taste
- Whole wheat buns for serving

Instructions:

1. In a slow cooker, combine barbecue sauce, chicken broth, brown sugar, paprika, garlic powder, onion powder, salt, and pepper.
2. Add chicken breasts to the slow cooker and coat them with the sauce mixture.
3. Cover and cook on low heat for 6-7 hours or until the chicken is tender and can be easily shredded.
4. Shred the chicken using two forks and mix it with the sauce.
5. Serve the BBQ pulled chicken on whole wheat buns.

Beef and Broccoli

Ingredients:

- 1 pound flank steak, thinly sliced
- 2 cups broccoli florets
- 1/4 cup low-sodium soy sauce
- 2 tablespoons brown sugar
- 2 cloves garlic, minced
- 1 teaspoon grated ginger
- 2 tablespoons vegetable oil
- Sesame seeds for garnish

- Cooked brown rice for serving

Instructions:

1. In a bowl, whisk together soy sauce, brown sugar, minced garlic, and grated ginger.
2. Heat vegetable oil in a large skillet or wok over high heat.
3. Add thinly sliced flank steak and stir-fry until browned. Remove from the skillet.
4. In the same skillet, add broccoli florets and stir-fry for a few minutes until they are tender-crisp.
5. Return the beef to the skillet and pour the sauce over it. Cook for another minute.
6. Serve over cooked brown rice and garnish with sesame seeds.

Roasted Vegetable Lasagna

Ingredients:

- 12 lasagna noodles, cooked and drained
- 2 cups ricotta cheese
- 2 cups shredded mozzarella cheese
- 1 cup grated Parmesan cheese

- 2 cups mixed roasted vegetables (e.g., bell peppers, zucchini, eggplant)
- 2 cups marinara sauce
- 1 teaspoon dried basil
- 1 teaspoon dried oregano
- Salt and pepper to taste

Instructions:

1. Preheat your oven to 350°F (175°C).
2. In a bowl, mix together ricotta cheese, 1 cup of mozzarella cheese, 1/2 cup of Parmesan cheese, dried basil, dried oregano, salt, and pepper.
3. In a 9x13-inch baking dish, spread a layer of marinara sauce.
4. Layer 4 cooked lasagna noodles on top of the sauce.
5. Spread half of the cheese mixture over the noodles, followed by half of the roasted vegetables.
6. Repeat the layers: sauce, noodles, cheese mixture, and roasted vegetables.
7. Top with the remaining 4 lasagna noodles, sauce, and the remaining mozzarella and Parmesan cheeses.

8. Cover with foil and bake for 30 minutes, then remove the foil and bake for an additional 15 minutes or until the lasagna is bubbly and golden.

Spinach Stuffed Chicken

Ingredients:

- 4 boneless, skinless chicken breasts
- 2 cups fresh spinach leaves
- 1/2 cup low-fat feta cheese
- 2 cloves garlic, minced
- 1 teaspoon dried basil
- 1 teaspoon dried oregano
- Salt and pepper to taste
- Olive oil for cooking

Instructions:

1. Preheat your oven to 375°F (190°C).
2. In a bowl, mix together fresh spinach leaves, low-fat feta cheese, minced garlic, dried basil, dried oregano, salt, and pepper.
3. Cut a pocket into each chicken breast without cutting all the way through.

4. Stuff each chicken breast with the spinach and feta mixture.

5. Heat olive oil in an ovenproof skillet over medium-high heat.

6. Brown the stuffed chicken breasts on both sides, then transfer the skillet to the oven.

7. Roast for 20-25 minutes or until the chicken is cooked through.

Vegetable Curry with Brown Rice

Ingredients:

- 2 cups mixed vegetables (e.g., carrots, bell peppers, cauliflower)
- 1 can (14 oz) chickpeas, drained and rinsed
- 1 onion, chopped
- 2 cloves garlic, minced
- 1 can (14 oz) diced tomatoes
- 1 can (14 oz) coconut milk
- 2 tablespoons curry powder
- 1 teaspoon ground turmeric
- Salt and pepper to taste
- Cooked brown rice for serving

Instructions:

1. In a large skillet or saucepan, sauté chopped onion and minced garlic until fragrant.

2. Add mixed vegetables and cook for a few minutes until they begin to soften.

3. Stir in chickpeas, diced tomatoes, coconut milk, curry powder, ground turmeric, salt, and pepper.

4. Simmer for 15-20 minutes until the vegetables are tender and the curry thickens.

5. Serve over cooked brown rice.

Chapter 5: Snacks and Appetizers

In Chapter 5, we delve into the world of delightful snacks and appetizers, perfect for satisfying your cravings while adhering to a low-potassium renal diet. These recipes are designed to not only tantalize your taste buds but also support your kidney health. Let's explore a variety of flavors and textures that will keep your snacking experience exciting.

Cucumber Slices with Hummus

Ingredients:

- 1 cucumber, thinly sliced
- 1/2 cup of your favorite hummus

Instructions:

1. Wash and slice the cucumber into thin rounds.
2. Serve the cucumber slices with a generous dollop of hummus for a refreshing and crunchy snack.

Guacamole and Salsa

Ingredients:

- 2 ripe avocados, peeled and mashed
- 1 tomato, diced
- 1/2 red onion, finely chopped
- 1/4 cup fresh cilantro, chopped
- Juice of 1 lime
- Salt and pepper to taste
- Your favorite low-sodium salsa

Instructions:

1. In a bowl, combine mashed avocados, diced tomato, chopped onion, cilantro, lime juice, salt, and pepper. Mix well.
2. Serve your homemade guacamole with a side of low-sodium salsa and enjoy with whole-grain tortilla chips or veggie sticks.

Baked Sweet Potato Fries

Ingredients:

- 2 sweet potatoes, cut into fries

- 1 tablespoon olive oil
- 1/2 teaspoon paprika
- 1/2 teaspoon garlic powder
- Salt and pepper to taste

Instructions:

1. Preheat your oven to 425°F (220°C).
2. In a bowl, toss sweet potato fries with olive oil, paprika, garlic powder, salt, and pepper.
3. Spread the fries in a single layer on a baking sheet.
4. Bake for 20-25 minutes or until they are golden and crispy. Flip them halfway through for even cooking.

Popcorn with Herbs

Ingredients:

- 1/2 cup popcorn kernels
- 2 tablespoons melted butter or olive oil
- 1 teaspoon dried rosemary
- 1/2 teaspoon dried thyme
- Salt to taste

Instructions:

1. Pop the popcorn kernels according to the package instructions.

2. In a large bowl, drizzle melted butter or olive oil over the popcorn.

3. Sprinkle dried rosemary, thyme, and salt over the popcorn and toss to coat evenly.

Greek Yogurt Dip with Veggies

Ingredients:

- 1 cup Greek yogurt
- 1 teaspoon lemon juice
- 1/2 teaspoon dried dill
- Assorted fresh vegetables for dipping (carrots, cucumber, bell peppers, etc.)

Instructions:

1. In a bowl, combine Greek yogurt, lemon juice, and dried dill. Mix until well combined.

2. Wash and prepare your choice of fresh vegetables for dipping.

3. Serve the Greek yogurt dip alongside the veggies for a creamy and nutritious snack.

Rice Cakes with Almond Butter

Ingredients:

- 2 rice cakes
- 2 tablespoons almond butter
- Sliced bananas (optional)

Instructions:

1. Spread almond butter evenly on each rice cake.
2. If desired, add sliced bananas on top.
3. Enjoy this quick and satisfying snack that combines crunch with creaminess.

Veggie Spring Rolls

Ingredients:

- 8 rice paper wrappers
- 1 cup shredded lettuce
- 1 cup thinly sliced cucumber
- 1 cup shredded carrots

- Fresh mint leaves (optional)
- Dipping sauce of your choice (low-sodium soy sauce, peanut sauce, or sweet chili sauce)

Instructions:

1. Fill a shallow dish with warm water.
2. Dip one rice paper wrapper into the water until it becomes pliable (usually about 10-15 seconds).
3. Lay the softened wrapper flat on a clean surface.
4. Place a small amount of lettuce, cucumber, carrots, and mint leaves (if using) in the center.
5. Fold in the sides of the wrapper and roll it up tightly.
6. Repeat with the remaining wrappers and filling.
7. Serve with your preferred dipping sauce.

Stuffed Mushrooms

Ingredients:

- 12 large mushrooms, cleaned and stems removed
- 1/2 cup low-fat cream cheese
- 1/4 cup grated Parmesan cheese
- 2 cloves garlic, minced
- 1 tablespoon fresh parsley, chopped

- Salt and pepper to taste

Instructions:

1. Preheat your oven to 350°F (175°C).

2. In a bowl, mix cream cheese, Parmesan cheese, minced garlic, chopped parsley, salt, and pepper until well combined.

3. Stuff each mushroom cap with the cream cheese mixture.

4. Arrange stuffed mushrooms on a baking sheet and bake for 15-20 minutes until the mushrooms are tender and the filling is lightly browned.

Cottage Cheese with Berries

Ingredients:

- 1/2 cup low-fat cottage cheese
- Mixed berries (e.g., strawberries, blueberries, raspberries)

Instructions:

1. Spoon the cottage cheese into a bowl.

2. Top with a generous serving of mixed berries for a delightful blend of creaminess and fruity sweetness.

Baked Parmesan Zucchini Chips

Ingredients:

- 2 medium-sized zucchinis, thinly sliced
- 1/2 cup grated Parmesan cheese
- 1/2 teaspoon garlic powder
- Salt and pepper to taste
- Olive oil spray

Instructions:

1. Preheat your oven to 425°F (220°C).
2. In a bowl, combine grated Parmesan cheese, garlic powder, salt, and pepper.
3. Place zucchini slices on a baking sheet and lightly spray them with olive oil.
4. Sprinkle the Parmesan mixture evenly over the zucchini slices.
5. Bake for about 20-25 minutes, or until the zucchini chips are golden and crispy.

Fruit Kabobs

Ingredients:

- Assorted fruits (e.g., melon, pineapple, grapes, strawberries)
- Wooden skewers

Instructions:

1. Wash and cut the fruits into bite-sized pieces.
2. Thread the fruit pieces onto wooden skewers in any desired pattern.
3. Arrange the fruit kabobs on a platter for a colorful and refreshing snack.

Spinach Artichoke Dip

Ingredients:

- 1 cup chopped spinach (thawed and drained if using frozen)
- 1 cup canned artichoke hearts, chopped
- 1 cup low-fat Greek yogurt
- 1/2 cup grated Parmesan cheese
- 1/2 cup low-fat mayonnaise

- 1/2 teaspoon garlic powder

- Salt and pepper to taste

Instructions:

1. In a bowl, combine chopped spinach, chopped artichoke hearts, Greek yogurt, Parmesan cheese, mayonnaise, garlic powder, salt, and pepper. Mix until well blended.

2. Transfer the mixture to an oven-safe dish and bake at 350°F (175°C) for about 20-25 minutes, or until bubbly and lightly browned.

3. Serve with whole-grain crackers or veggie sticks for dipping.

Roasted Red Pepper and Walnut Dip

Ingredients:

- 2 red bell peppers, roasted, peeled, and seeded

- 1/2 cup walnuts, toasted

- 2 cloves garlic, minced

- 2 tablespoons olive oil

- 1 teaspoon lemon juice

- Salt and pepper to taste

Instructions:

1. Place roasted red peppers, toasted walnuts, minced garlic, olive oil, lemon juice, salt, and pepper in a blender or food processor.

2. Blend until you achieve a smooth and creamy consistency.

3. Serve as a dip with vegetable sticks or whole-grain crackers.

Celery and Peanut Butter

Ingredients:

- Celery sticks
- Natural peanut butter (low-sodium and unsweetened)

Instructions:

1. Spread a thin layer of natural peanut butter on celery sticks.

2. The classic combination of crunchy celery and creamy peanut butter makes for a satisfying and simple snack.

Edamame

Ingredients:

- Edamame pods
- Sea salt (optional)

Instructions:

1. Steam or boil the edamame pods until tender, about 3-5 minutes.
2. Drain and sprinkle with sea salt if desired.
3. Enjoy these protein-packed soybean pods as a wholesome and nutritious snack.

Caprese Skewers

Ingredients:

- Cherry tomatoes
- Fresh mozzarella balls
- Fresh basil leaves
- Balsamic glaze (low-sodium)

Instructions:

1. Thread cherry tomatoes, mozzarella balls, and fresh basil leaves onto skewers.

2. Drizzle with a touch of balsamic glaze for a burst of Italian-inspired flavors.

Apple Slices with Cinnamon

Ingredients:

- Apple slices
- Ground cinnamon

Instructions:

1. Slice apples into thin rounds or wedges.

2. Sprinkle ground cinnamon over the apple slices for a sweet and slightly spicy treat.

Mini Quiches

Ingredients:

- 6 large eggs
- 1/2 cup milk (low-fat)
- Salt and pepper to taste

- Chopped vegetables (e.g., bell peppers, spinach, mushrooms)
- Shredded low-fat cheese (optional)

Instructions:

1. Preheat your oven to 350°F (175°C).
2. In a bowl, whisk together eggs, milk, salt, and pepper.
3. Grease a muffin tin and distribute chopped vegetables (and cheese if using) evenly among the cups.
4. Pour the egg mixture over the vegetables in each cup.
5. Bake for approximately 20-25 minutes or until the quiches are set and slightly golden.

Chapter 6: Desserts

Welcome to the sweet finale of your culinary journey through the Low-Potassium Renal Diet Cookbook. In Chapter 6, we present delightful dessert recipes that not only satisfy your sweet tooth but also adhere to your dietary restrictions. Let's dive into these mouthwatering creations that bring joy to your tastebuds without compromising your health.

Banana Ice Cream

Ingredients:

- 2 ripe bananas
- 1/4 cup almond milk
- 1 tsp vanilla extract

Instructions:

1. Peel and slice the bananas, then freeze them until solid.
2. Blend the frozen bananas, almond milk, and vanilla extract until smooth.

3. Enjoy immediately or freeze for a firmer texture.

Baked Apples

Ingredients:

- 4 apples (Granny Smith or Fuji work well)
- 1/4 cup chopped walnuts
- 1/4 cup raisins
- 1 tsp cinnamon
- 1 tbsp honey (optional)

Instructions:

1. Preheat your oven to 350°F (175°C).
2. Core the apples and remove some of the flesh to create a well.
3. Mix the walnuts, raisins, cinnamon, and honey (if using) in a bowl.
4. Stuff each apple with the mixture.
5. Place the apples in a baking dish, add a little water to the bottom, and cover with foil.
6. Bake for 30-40 minutes or until apples are tender.

Chocolate Avocado Mousse

Ingredients:

- 2 ripe avocados
- 1/4 cup cocoa powder
- 1/4 cup honey
- 1 tsp vanilla extract

Instructions:

1. Blend avocados, cocoa powder, honey, and vanilla extract until smooth.
2. Chill in the refrigerator for at least 30 minutes.
3. Serve with fresh berries.

Rice Pudding with Cinnamon

Ingredients:

- 1 cup cooked white rice
- 2 cups milk (or non-dairy milk)
- 1/4 cup sugar
- 1 tsp vanilla extract
- 1/2 tsp ground cinnamon

Instructions:

1. Combine cooked rice, milk, sugar, vanilla extract, and cinnamon in a saucepan.
2. Cook over medium heat, stirring until the mixture thickens.
3. Remove from heat and let it cool before serving.

Berry Parfait

Ingredients:

- 1 cup low-potassium granola
- 1 cup mixed berries (strawberries, blueberries, raspberries)
- 1 cup Greek yogurt

Instructions:

1. Layer a glass or bowl with granola, followed by yogurt and mixed berries.
2. Repeat the layers.
3. Finish with a sprinkle of granola on top.

Poached Pears

Ingredients:

- 4 ripe pears
- 2 cups water
- 1/2 cup sugar
- 1 cinnamon stick

Instructions:

1. Peel and core the pears, leaving the stems intact.
2. In a pot, combine water, sugar, and the cinnamon stick. Bring to a simmer.
3. Add pears and simmer for about 20 minutes or until tender.
4. Remove pears and let the syrup cool.
5. Drizzle syrup over the pears before serving.

Chia Seed Pudding

Ingredients:

- 1/4 cup chia seeds
- 1 cup almond milk
- 1 tsp vanilla extract

- Fresh fruit for topping

Instructions:

1. Mix chia seeds, almond milk, and vanilla extract in a bowl.
2. Stir well and refrigerate for at least 4 hours or overnight, stirring occasionally.
3. Serve with fresh fruit.

Sorbet Trio

Ingredients:

- 1 cup frozen mango chunks
- 1 cup frozen raspberry
- 1 cup frozen pineapple
- 1/4 cup honey (optional)

Instructions:

1. Blend each frozen fruit separately until smooth.
2. Sweeten with honey if desired.
3. Layer the three sorbets in a glass or bowl.
4. Enjoy a burst of fruity flavors.

Lemon Bars

Ingredients:

- 1 cup low-potassium graham cracker crumbs
- 2 tbsp melted butter
- 1 cup lemon juice
- 1 cup sugar
- 3 large eggs

Instructions:

1. Mix graham cracker crumbs and melted butter, press into a baking dish.
2. In a separate bowl, whisk together lemon juice, sugar, and eggs.
3. Pour lemon mixture over the crust.
4. Bake at 350°F (175°C) for 25-30 minutes.
5. Let it cool and cut into bars.

Pumpkin Pie Smoothie

Ingredients:

- 1/2 cup canned pumpkin puree
- 1 cup almond milk

- 1 tsp pumpkin pie spice

- 1 tbsp maple syrup (optional)

- Ice cubes

Instructions:

1. Blend pumpkin puree, almond milk, pumpkin pie spice, and maple syrup (if using) until smooth.

2. Add ice cubes and blend again until creamy.

Strawberry Shortcake

Ingredients:

- 4 low-potassium shortcake biscuits

- 2 cups sliced strawberries

- 1 cup whipped cream (or whipped coconut cream)

Instructions:

1. Slice shortcake biscuits in half horizontally.

2. Layer strawberries and whipped cream between the biscuit halves.

3. Top with additional strawberries and a dollop of whipped cream.

Oatmeal Raisin Cookies

Ingredients:

- 1 cup rolled oats
- 1/2 cup mashed bananas
- 1/4 cup raisins
- 1/4 cup chopped walnuts
- 1/4 tsp cinnamon

Instructions:

1. Mix rolled oats, mashed bananas, raisins, chopped walnuts, and cinnamon in a bowl.
2. Drop spoonfuls of dough onto a baking sheet.
3. Bake at 350°F (175°C) for 15-20 minutes or until golden brown.

Mixed Berry Crisp

Ingredients:

- 3 cups mixed berries
- 1/2 cup low-potassium granola
- 2 tbsp honey (optional)

Instructions:

1. Place mixed berries in a baking dish.
2. Sprinkle granola on top.
3. Drizzle with honey (if desired).
4. Bake at 350°F (175°C) for 20-25 minutes or until bubbly.

Angel Food Cake with Berries

Ingredients:

- 1 store-bought angel food cake (low-potassium)
- 2 cups mixed berries
- 1 cup whipped cream (or whipped coconut cream)

Instructions:

1. Slice the angel food cake into serving portions.
2. Top each slice with mixed berries and a dollop of whipped cream.

Coconut Macaroons

Ingredients:

- 2 cups shredded unsweetened coconut

- 3/4 cup sweetened condensed milk (low-potassium)
- 1 tsp vanilla extract
- 2 egg whites
- Pinch of salt

Instructions:

1. In a bowl, combine shredded coconut, sweetened condensed milk, and vanilla extract.
2. In a separate bowl, whip egg whites with a pinch of salt until stiff peaks form.
3. Gently fold whipped egg whites into the coconut mixture.
4. Drop spoonfuls of the mixture onto a baking sheet.
5. Bake at 325°F (160°C) for 20-25 minutes or until golden brown.

Chocolate Covered Strawberries

Ingredients:

- 12 fresh strawberries
- 1/2 cup dark chocolate chips (low-potassium)

Instructions:

1. Melt dark chocolate chips in a microwave-safe bowl, stirring every 30 seconds until smooth.
2. Dip each strawberry into the melted chocolate, coating them partially.
3. Place on a parchment-lined tray and refrigerate until the chocolate hardens.

Peach Cobbler

Ingredients:

- 4 cups sliced canned peaches (in juice, drained)
- 1 cup low-potassium baking mix
- 1/2 cup sugar
- 1/2 cup milk

Instructions:

1. Preheat oven to 350°F (175°C).
2. Spread peaches in a baking dish.
3. In a separate bowl, mix baking mix, sugar, and milk until a batter forms.
4. Pour the batter over the peaches.
5. Bake for 30-35 minutes or until golden brown.

Almond Joy Bites

Ingredients:

- 1 cup unsweetened shredded coconut
- 1/2 cup almond butter
- 1/4 cup honey
- 1/4 cup dark chocolate chips (low-potassium)

Instructions:

1. Mix shredded coconut, almond butter, and honey in a bowl.
2. Roll the mixture into bite-sized balls.
3. Melt dark chocolate chips in a microwave-safe bowl.
4. Dip each ball into the melted chocolate, coating them partially.
5. Place on a parchment-lined tray and refrigerate until the chocolate hardens.

CONCLUSION

In this final chapter of the "Low-Potassium Renal Diet Cookbook," we reach the culmination of your journey towards embracing a healthier, kidney-friendly lifestyle. It's not just an ending; it's a new beginning filled with valuable insights and encouragement.

As you've ventured through the pages of this cookbook, you've discovered a world of delicious and nutritious low-potassium recipes designed specifically to support your renal health.

Final Thoughts and Encouragement:

Lastly, we'll leave you with heartfelt final thoughts and words of encouragement. Remember that your dedication to this journey is commendable, and every small step you take towards better kidney health is a victory. You're not alone on this path; there is a community of individuals just like you who are striving for a healthier life.

As you turn the page and close the "Low-Potassium Renal Diet Cookbook," know that this isn't the end—it's a continuation of your commitment to your well-being. Your kidneys will thank you for the care you've shown them, and your body will reap the rewards of a balanced and kidney-friendly diet. Embrace this conclusion as the launchpad for a healthier, happier you.

www.ingramcontent.com/pod-product-compliance
Lightning Source LLC
Chambersburg PA
CBHW070832260726

48660CB00005B/2023